# The Super Easy Vegetarian Cooking Guide

## Mouth-watering Vegetarian Recipes For Beginners

*Riley Bloom*

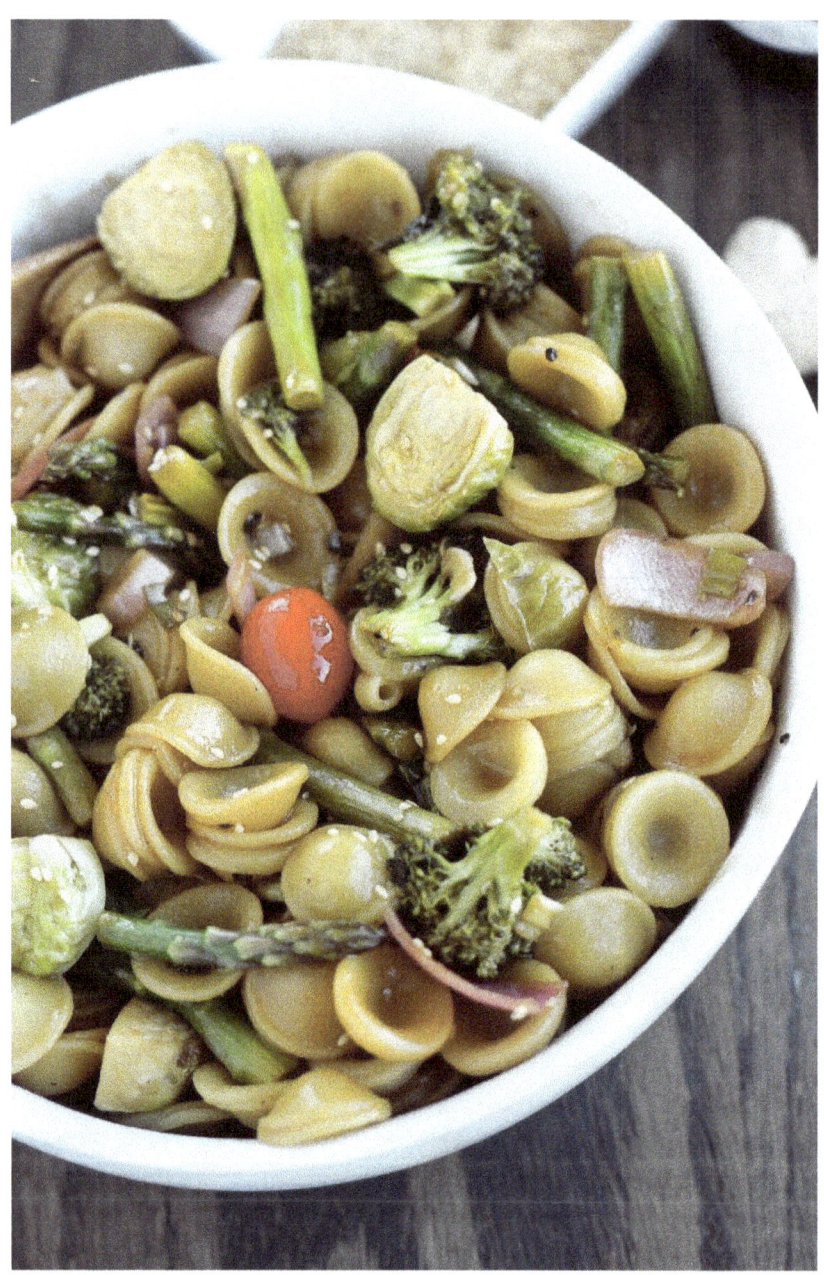

## © Copyright 2020 - All rights reserved.

The content contained within this book may not be reproduced, duplicated or transmitted without direct written permission from the author or the publisher.

Under no circumstances will any blame or legal responsibility be held against the publisher, or author, for any damages, reparation, or monetary loss due to the information contained within this book. Either directly or indirectly.

**Legal Notice:**

This book is copyright protected. This book is only for personal use. You cannot amend, distribute, sell, use, quote or paraphrase any part, or the content within this book, without the consent of the author or publisher.

**Disclaimer Notice:**

Please note the information contained within this document is for educational and entertainment purposes only. All effort has been executed to present accurate, up to date, and reliable, complete information. No warranties of any kind are declared or implied. Readers acknowledge that the author is not engaging in the rendering of legal, financial, medical or professional advice. The content within this book has been derived from various sources. Please consult a licensed professional before attempting any techniques outlined in this book.

By reading this document, the reader agrees that under no circumstances is the author responsible for any losses, direct or indirect, which are incurred as a result of the use of information contained within this document, including, but not limited to, — errors, omissions, or inaccuracies.

# Table of contents

Elbow Macaroni with Black and White Beans .................................................. 7

Fettuccini Green Olives and Parmesan Cheese............................................. 10

Spaghetti with Chorizo and Mozarella ........................................................ 13

Macaroni and Pepper Jack Cheese ............................................................. 15

Macaroni with Cream Cheese and Mozarella............................................... 17

Whole Wheat Macaroni With Mozzarella and Parmesan Cheese............... 19

Papardelle Pasta with Cheddar Cheese ...................................................... 22

Pasta Shells in Chimichurri Sauce with Cream Cheese ............................. 24

Spaghetti with Pepper Jack Cheese and Mozarella ................................... 26

Pasta with Pesto and Mozarella ................................................................. 28

Macaroni and Mozarella and Monterey Jack Cheese ................................. 31

Fettuccini with Pinto Beans and Cheddar Cheese ..................................... 33

Papardelle Pasta and Gouda Cheese........................................................... 35

Pasta Shells with Cheddar Cheese and Capers ..........................................37

Elbow Macaroni with Olives and Capers.................................................... 39

Elbow Macaroni with Crimini Mushrooms..................................................41

Papardelle Pasta and Oyster Mushroom and Vegan Chorizo ................... 43

Creamy Elbow Mac and Vegan Italian Sausage ......................................... 45

Pasta Shells with Tomato Sauce and Ricotta Cheese................................47

Papardelle Pasta with Ricotta Cheese........................................................ 49

Lima Beans with Quinoa ..............................................................................51

Vegetarian Brown Rice Burrito Bowl ............................................................. 54

Garbanzo Bean Burrito Bowl with Sun-dried Pesto ................................. 56

White Bean Vegetarian Burrito Bowl ............................................................ 58

Vegetarian Garbanzo Bean Burrito Bowl ..................................................... 59

White Bean and Ricotta Cheese Burrito Bowl ............................................ 62

Red Rice and Garbanzo Beans with Chimichurri Sauce .......................... 64

White Beans and Italian Sausage Burrito Bowl ......................................... 66

Smoky Red Rice with Garbanzo Beans ........................................................ 68

Vegan Chorizo Burrito Bowl ........................................................................... 70

Chimichurri Vegan Chorizo Burrito Bowl ................................................... 72

Smoky White Bean & White Rice Burrito Bowl ......................................... 74

Red Rice with Vegan Chorizo and Tomatoes ............................................. 76

White Bean & Vegan Chorizo Burrito ........................................................... 78

Red Rice with Vegan Chorizo ......................................................................... 80

Quinoa and Lima Bean Chili .......................................................................... 82

Tangy Pesto Chili ............................................................................................... 84

Vegan Burger and Lentils ................................................................................ 86

Slow Cooked Thai Mung Beans and Black Rice ........................................ 89

Quinoa with Beans ............................................................................................ 91

Smoky Brown Rice with Vegan Italian Sausage ........................................ 94

Dried Black Beans and Quinoa in Pesto ...................................................... 96

Vegetarian Meatballs and Quinoa ................................................................. 98

Slow Cooked Thai Black Rice with Mung Beans ..................................... 100

Red Rice and Vegetarian Meat Sausage with Jalapeno Pepper ............... 102

Spicy Brown Rice with Vegan Chorizo ...................................................... 104

Kidney Beans & Button Mushrooms with Pesto Sauce ........................... 106

# Elbow Macaroni with Black and White Beans

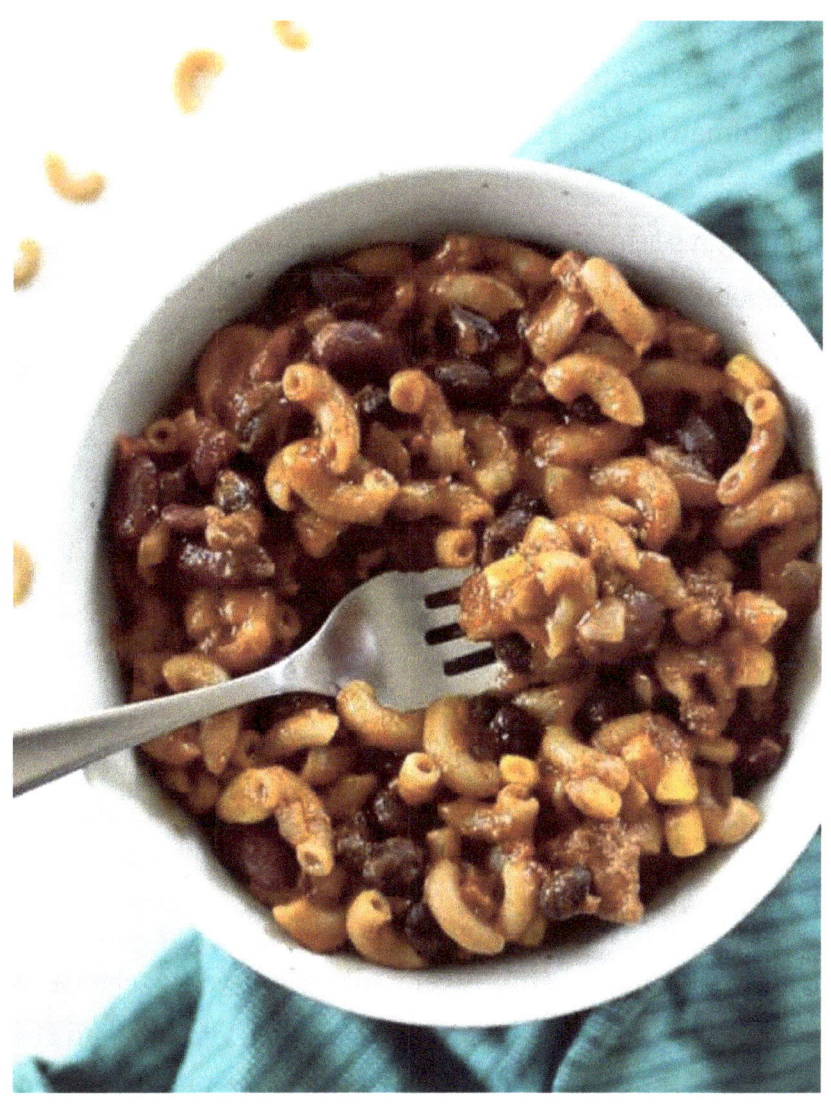

## Ingredients

1 red onion, medium chopped

1 green bell pepper chopped

15 ounce can white beans

15 ounce can black beans

28 ounce crushed tomatoes

2 tbsp. tomato paste

1 tsp. basil

1 tsp. Italian seasoning

½ teaspoon salt

1/8 teaspoon black pepper

2 cups vegetable stock

8 ounces whole wheat elbow macaroni pasta uncooked

1 ½ cups Vegan Cheese (Tofu Based)

Garnishing ingredients:

chopped green onions for serving

## Directions:

Put all of the ingredients except for pasta, vegan cheese, and garnishing ingredients in your slow cooker. Combine and cover. Cook on high heat for 4 hours or low heat for 7 hours.

Add the pasta and cooking on high heat for 18 minutes, or until pasta becomes al dente Add 1 cup of cheese and stir. Sprinkle with the remaining cheese and garnishing ingredients

# Fettuccini Green Olives and Parmesan Cheese

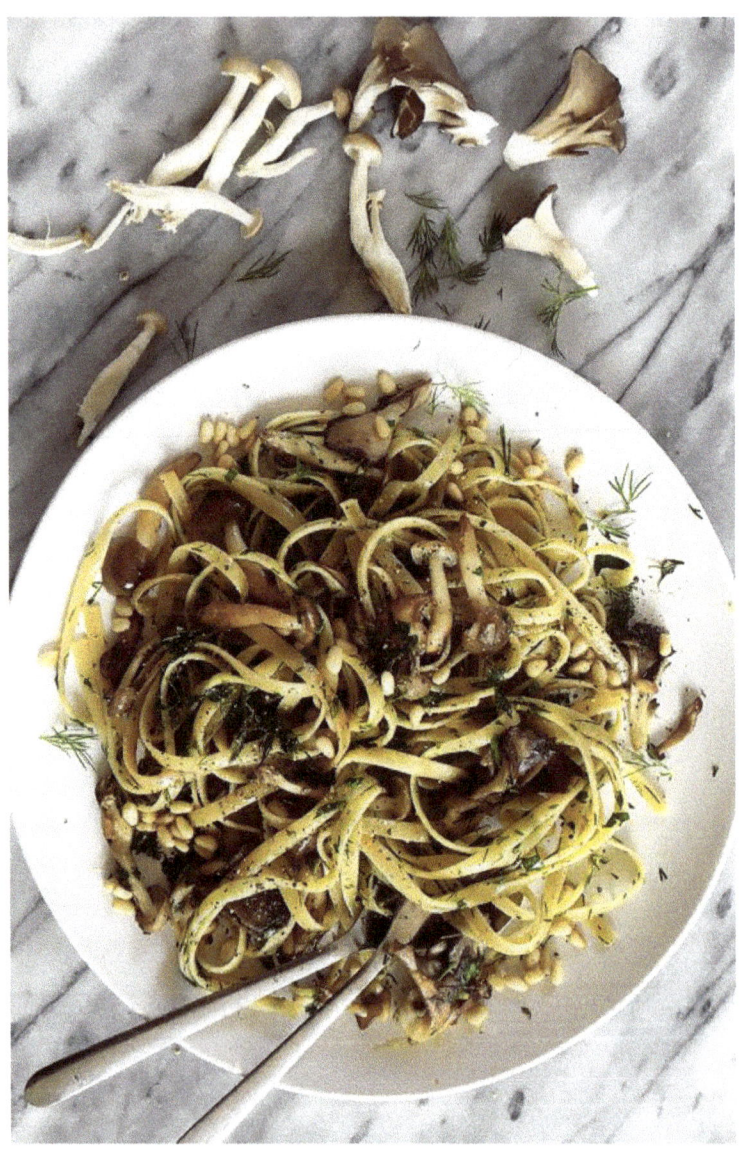

## Ingredients

1 red onion, medium chopped

1 green bell pepper chopped

15 ounce can fava beans, rinsed and drained

15 ounce can navy beans, rinsed and drained

28 ounce crushed tomatoes

1/4 cup green olives

2 tbsp. capers

½ teaspoon salt

1/8 teaspoon black pepper

2 cups vegetable stock

8 ounces fettuccini uncooked

1 ½ cups Parmesan Cheese

Garnishing ingredients:

chopped green onions for serving

## Directions:

Put all of the ingredients except for pasta, cheese, and garnishing ingredients in your slow cooker. Combine and cover. Cook on high heat for 4 hours or low heat for 7 hours.

Add the pasta and cooking on high heat for 18 minutes, or until pasta becomes al dente Add 1 cup of cheese and stir. Sprinkle with the remaining cheese and garnishing ingredients

# Spaghetti with Chorizo and Mozarella

**Ingredients**

1 red onion, medium chopped

1 green bell pepper chopped

15 ounce can kidney beans

15 ounce can great northern beans

28 ounce crushed tomatoes

1/4 cup vegan chorizos, coarsely chopped

1 tsp. dried thyme

½ teaspoon salt

1/8 teaspoon black pepper

2 cups vegetable stock

8 ounces spaghetti noodles uncooked

1 ½ cups Mozarella Cheese

Garnishing ingredients:

chopped green onions for serving

**Directions:**

Put all of the ingredients except for pasta, mozarella cheese, and garnishing ingredients in your slow cooker. Combine and cover. Cook on high heat for 4 hours or low heat for 7 hours. Add the pasta and cooking on high heat for 18 minutes, or until pasta becomes al dente Add 1 cup of cheese and stir. Sprinkle with the remaining mozarella cheese and garnishing ingredients

# Macaroni and Pepper Jack Cheese

## Ingredients

15 ounce can lima beans rinsed and drained

15 ounce can garbanzo beans rinsed and drained

28 ounce crushed tomatoes

4 tbsp. pesto

1 tsp. Italian seasoning

½ teaspoon salt

1/8 teaspoon black pepper

2 cups vegetable stock

8 ounces whole wheat elbow macaroni pasta uncooked

1 ½ cups Pepper Jack Cheese

<u>Garnishing ingredients:</u>

chopped green onions for serving

## Directions:

Put all of the ingredients except for pasta, cheese, and garnishing ingredients in your slow cooker. Combine and cover. Cook on high heat for 4 hours or low heat for 7 hours.

Add the pasta and cooking on high heat for 18 minutes, or until pasta becomes al dente Add 1 cup of cheese and stir. Sprinkle with the remaining cheese and garnishing ingredients

# Macaroni with Cream Cheese and Mozarella

## Ingredients

1 red onion, medium chopped

1 green bell pepper chopped

15 ounce can kidney beans

15 ounce can lima beans

28 ounce crushed tomatoes

3 ounces vegan mozzarella

1 tsp. Italian seasoning

½ teaspoon salt

1/8 teaspoon black pepper

2 cups vegetable stock

8 ounces whole wheat elbow macaroni pasta uncooked

1 ½ cups Cream Cheese

<u>Garnishing ingredients:</u>

chopped green onions for serving

## Directions:

Put all of the ingredients except for pasta, vegan cheese, and garnishing ingredients in your slow cooker. Combine and cover.

Cook on high heat for 4 hours or low heat for 7 hours. Add the pasta and cooking on high heat for 18 minutes, or until pasta becomes al dente Add 1 cup of cheese and stir. Sprinkle with the remaining cheese and garnishing ingredients

# Whole Wheat Macaroni With Mozzarella and Parmesan Cheese

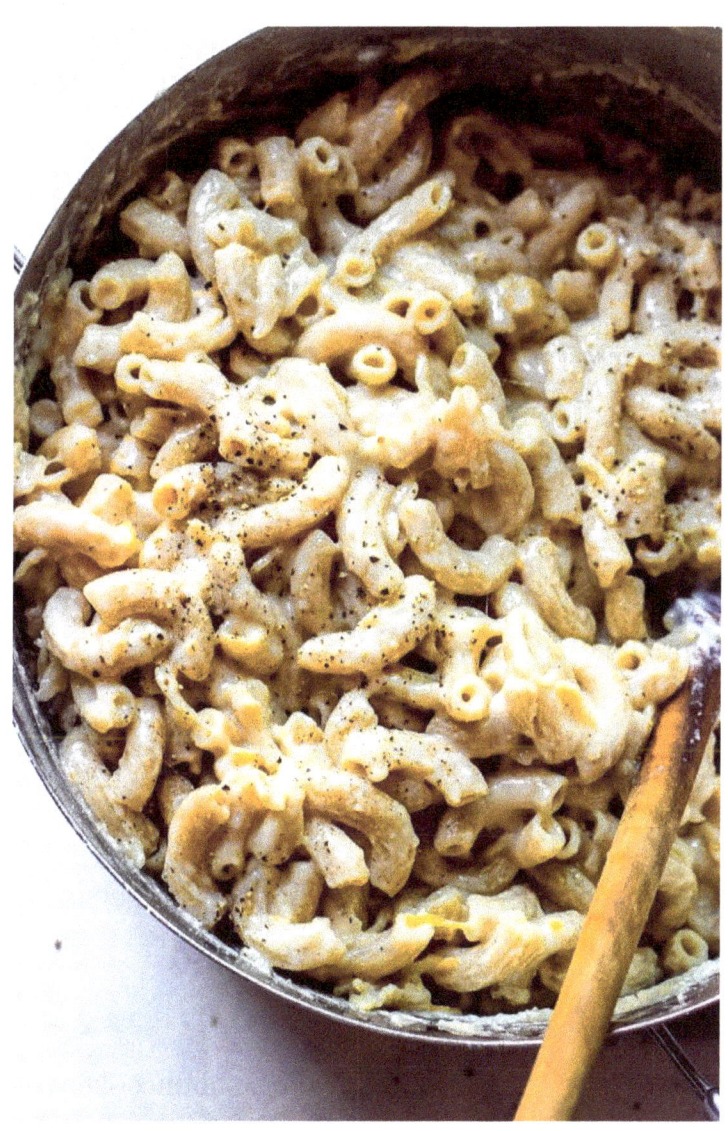

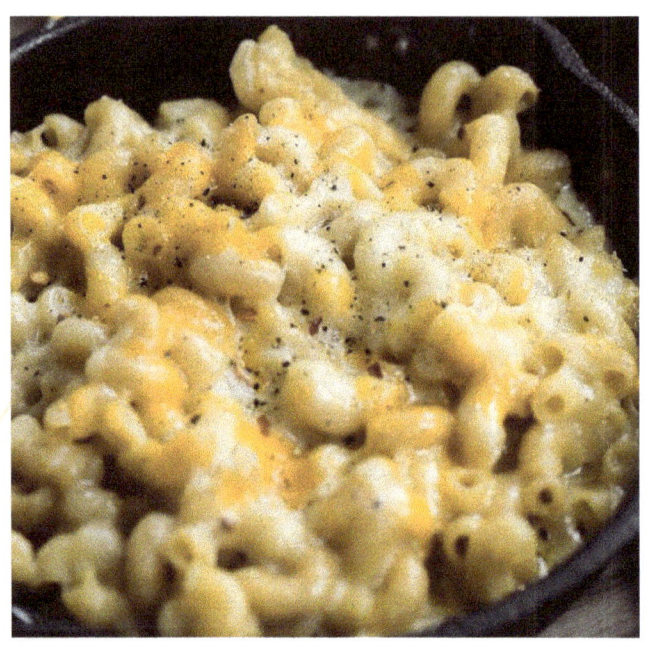

**Ingredients**

1 red onion, medium chopped

1 green bell pepper chopped

28 ounce crushed tomatoes

4 tbsp. vegan cream cheese

1 tsp. herbs de Provence

½ teaspoon salt

1/8 teaspoon black pepper

2 cups vegetable stock

8 ounces whole wheat elbow macaroni pasta uncooked

1 cups Mozarella Cheese

½ cup parmesan cheese

Garnishing ingredients:

chopped green onions for serving

**Directions:**

Put all of the ingredients except for pasta, vegan cheese, and garnishing ingredients in your slow cooker. Combine and cover. Cook on high heat for 4 hours or low heat for 7 hours. Add the pasta and cooking on high heat for 18 minutes, or until pasta becomes al dente Add 1 cup of mozzarella cheese and stir. Sprinkle with the remaining parmesan cheese and garnishing ingredients

# Papardelle Pasta with Cheddar Cheese

## Ingredients

1 red onion, medium chopped

1 green bell pepper chopped

15 ounce can fava beans, rinsed and drained

15 ounce can navy beans, rinsed and drained

28 ounce crushed tomatoes

4 tbsp. pesto

1 tsp. Italian seasoning

½ teaspoon salt

1/8 teaspoon black pepper

2 cups vegetable stock

8 ounces pappardelle pasta uncooked

1 ¼ cups Mozarella Cheese

¼ cup Cheddar Cheese

<u>Garnishing ingredients:</u>

chopped green onions for serving

## Directions:

Put all of the ingredients except for pasta, vegan cheese, and garnishing ingredients in your slow cooker. Combine and cover.

Cook on high heat for 4 hours or low heat for 7 hours. Add the pasta and cooking on high heat for 18 minutes, or until pasta becomes al dente Add 1 cup of mozzarella cheese and stir. Sprinkle with the remaining cheese and garnishing ingredients

# Pasta Shells in Chimichurri Sauce with Cream Cheese

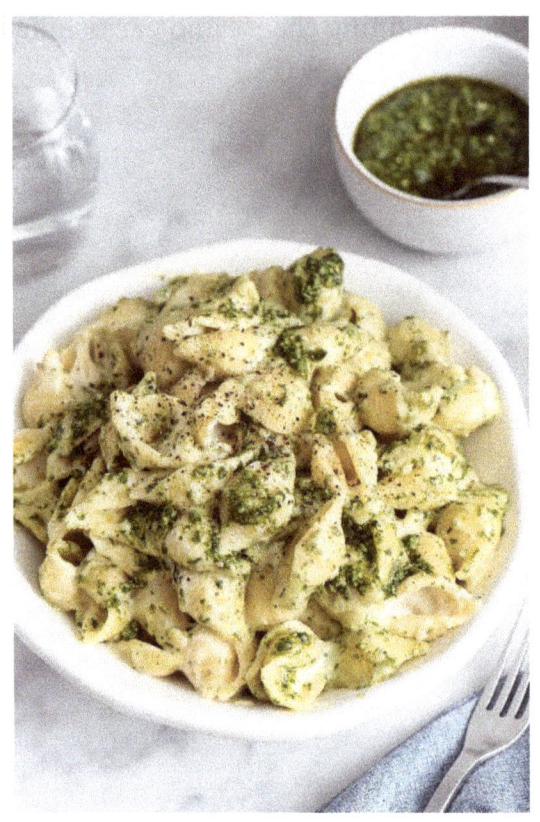

## Ingredients

5 jalapeno peppers

4 tbsp. chimichurri sauce

1/2 tsp. cayenne pepper

½ teaspoon salt

1/8 teaspoon black pepper

2 cups vegetable stock

8 ounces pasta shells uncooked

1 ½ cups Cream Cheese

Garnishing ingredients:

chopped green onions for serving

**Directions:**

Put all of the ingredients except for pasta, vegan cheese, and garnishing ingredients in your slow cooker. Combine and cover. Cook on high heat for 4 hours or low heat for 7 hours. Add the pasta and cooking on high heat for 18 minutes, or until pasta becomes al dente Add 1 cup of cheese and stir. Sprinkle with the remaining cheese and garnishing ingredients

# Spaghetti with Pepper Jack Cheese and Mozarella

## Ingredients

1 red onion, medium chopped

1 green bell pepper chopped

14 ounce crushed green tomatoes

14 ounce crushed tomatoes

3 ounces vegan mozzarella

1 tsp. Italian seasoning

½ teaspoon salt

1/8 teaspoon black pepper

2 cups vegetable stock

8 ounces spaghetti noodles uncooked

1 ½ cups Pepper Jack Cheese , shredded

<u>Garnishing ingredients:</u>

chopped green onions for serving

## Directions:

Put all of the ingredients except for pasta, vegan cheese, and garnishing ingredients in your slow cooker. Combine and cover. Cook on high heat for 4 hours or low heat for 7 hours. Add the

pasta and cooking on high heat for 18 minutes, or until pasta becomes al dente Add 1 cup of pepper jack cheese and stir. Sprinkle with the remaining pepper jack cheese and garnishing ingredients

# Pasta with Pesto and Mozarella

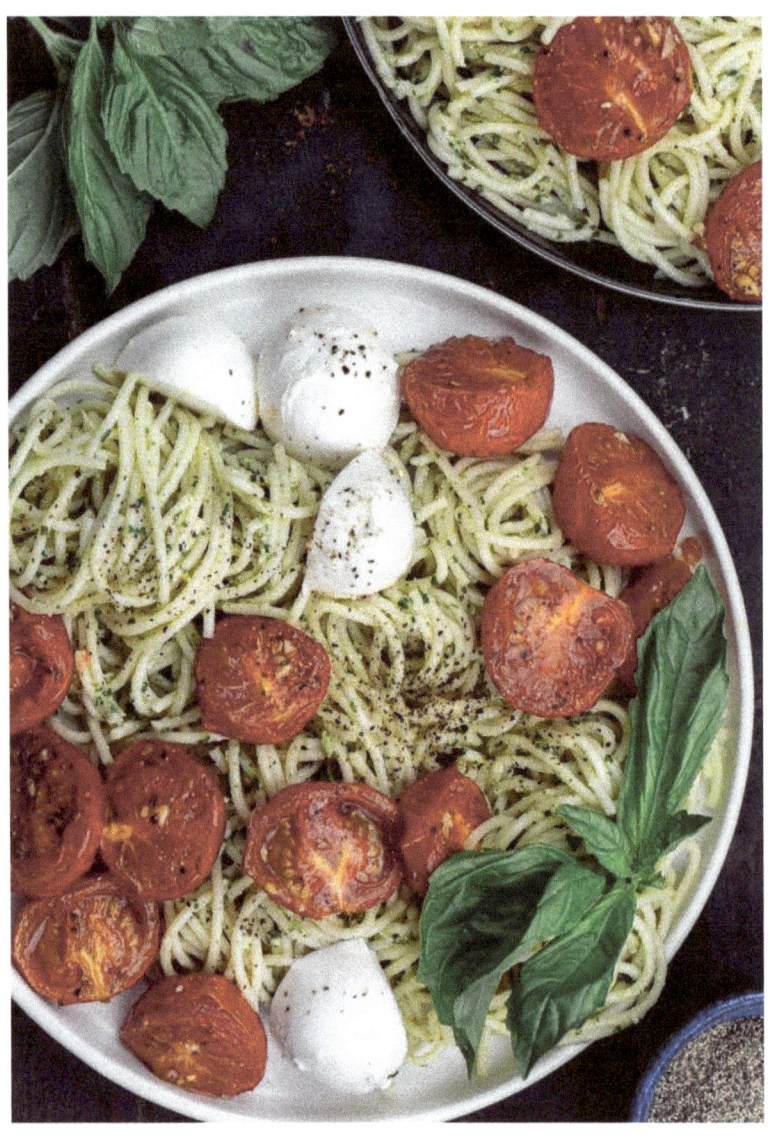

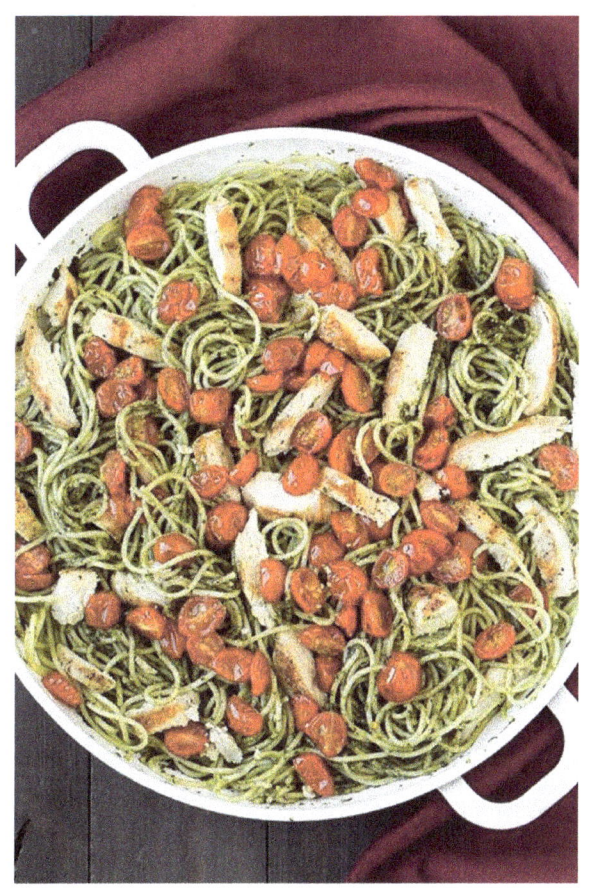

**Ingredients**

1 red onion, medium chopped

1 green bell pepper chopped

15 ounce can lima beans, rinsed and drained

15 ounce can soy beans, rinsed and drained

28 ounce crushed tomatoes

4 tbsp. pesto

1 tsp. Italian seasoning

½ teaspoon salt

1/8 teaspoon black pepper

2 cups vegetable stock

8 ounces penne pasta uncooked

1 ½ cups Mozarella Cheese

Garnishing ingredients:

chopped green onions for serving

**Directions:**

Put all of the ingredients except for pasta, vegan cheese, and garnishing ingredients in your slow cooker. Combine and cover. Cook on high heat for 4 hours or low heat for 7 hours. Add the pasta and cooking on high heat for 18 minutes, or until pasta becomes al dente Add 1 cup of cheese and stir. Sprinkle with the remaining cheese and garnishing ingredients

# Macaroni and Mozarella and Monterey Jack Cheese

## Ingredients

1 yellow onion, medium chopped

28 ounce crushed tomatoes

1/4 cup vegan chorizos, coarsely chopped

1 tsp. dried thyme

½ teaspoon salt

1/8 teaspoon black pepper

2 cups vegetable stock

8 ounces whole wheat elbow macaroni pasta uncooked

1 ½ cups Mozarella Cheese

½ cup Monterey Jack Cheese

Garnishing ingredients:

chopped green onions for serving

## Directions:

Put all of the ingredients except for pasta, vegan cheese, and garnishing ingredients in your slow cooker. Combine and cover. Cook on high heat for 4 hours or low heat for 7 hours.

Add the pasta and cooking on high heat for 18 minutes, or until pasta becomes al dente Add 1 cup of cheese and stir. Sprinkle with the remaining vegan cheese and garnishing ingredients

# Fettuccini with Pinto Beans and Cheddar Cheese

## Ingredients

1 red onion, medium chopped

1 green bell pepper chopped

8 cloves garlic, minced

28 ounce crushed tomatoes

4 tbsp. vegan cream cheese

1 tsp. herbs de Provence

½ teaspoon salt

1/8 teaspoon black pepper

2 cups vegetable stock

8 ounces fettuccini uncooked

1 ½ cups Cheddar Cheese

<u>Garnishing ingredients:</u>

chopped green onions for serving

## Directions:

Put all of the ingredients except for pasta, vegan cheese, and garnishing ingredients in your slow cooker. Combine and cover. Cook on high heat for 4 hours or low heat for 7 hours. Add the

pasta and cooking on high heat for 18 minutes, or until pasta becomes al dente Add 1 cup of cheese and stir. Sprinkle with the remaining cheese and garnishing ingredients

# Papardelle Pasta and Gouda Cheese

## Ingredients

1 yellow onion, medium chopped

1 red bell pepper, chopped

28 ounce crushed green tomatoes

2 tbsp. tomato paste

1 tsp. basil

1 tsp. Italian seasoning

½ teaspoon salt

1/8 teaspoon black pepper

2 cups vegetable stock

8 ounces pappardelle pasta uncooked

1 ½ cups gouda cheese

<u>Garnishing ingredients:</u>

chopped green onions for serving

## Directions:

Put all of the ingredients except for pasta, vegan cheese, and garnishing ingredients in your slow cooker. Combine and cover. Cook on high heat for 4 hours or low heat for 7 hours.

Add the pasta and cooking on high heat for 18 minutes, or until pasta becomes al dente Add 1 cup of cheese and stir. Sprinkle with the remaining gouda cheese and garnishing ingredients

# Pasta Shells with Cheddar Cheese and Capers

## Ingredients

1 red onion, medium chopped

1 green bell pepper chopped

¼ cup capers, drained

4 tbsp. chimichurri sauce

1/2 tsp. cayenne pepper

½ teaspoon salt

1/8 teaspoon black pepper

2 cups vegetable stock

8 ounces pasta shells uncooked

1 ½ cups Cheddar Cheese

<u>Garnishing ingredients:</u>

chopped green onions for serving

## Directions:

Put all of the ingredients except for pasta, vegan cheese, and garnishing ingredients in your slow cooker. Combine and cover. Cook on high heat for 4 hours or low heat for 7 hours.

Add the pasta and cooking on high heat for 18 minutes, or until pasta becomes al dente Add 1 cup of cheese and stir. Sprinkle with the remaining cheese and garnishing ingredients

# Elbow Macaroni with Olives and Capers

## Ingredients

1 red onion, medium chopped

15 ounce can button mushrooms

28 ounce crushed tomatoes

1/4 cup green olives

2 tbsp. capers

½ teaspoon salt

1/8 teaspoon black pepper

2 cups vegetable stock

8 ounces whole wheat elbow macaroni pasta uncooked

1 ½ cups Vegan Cheese (Tofu Based)

Garnishing ingredients:

chopped green onions for serving

## Directions:

Put all of the ingredients except for pasta, cheese, and garnishing ingredients in your slow cooker. Combine and cover. Cook on high heat for 4 hours or low heat for 7 hours.

Add the pasta and cooking on high heat for 18 minutes, or until pasta becomes al dente Add 1 cup of cheese and stir. Sprinkle with the remaining vegan cheese and garnishing ingredients

# Elbow Macaroni with Crimini Mushrooms

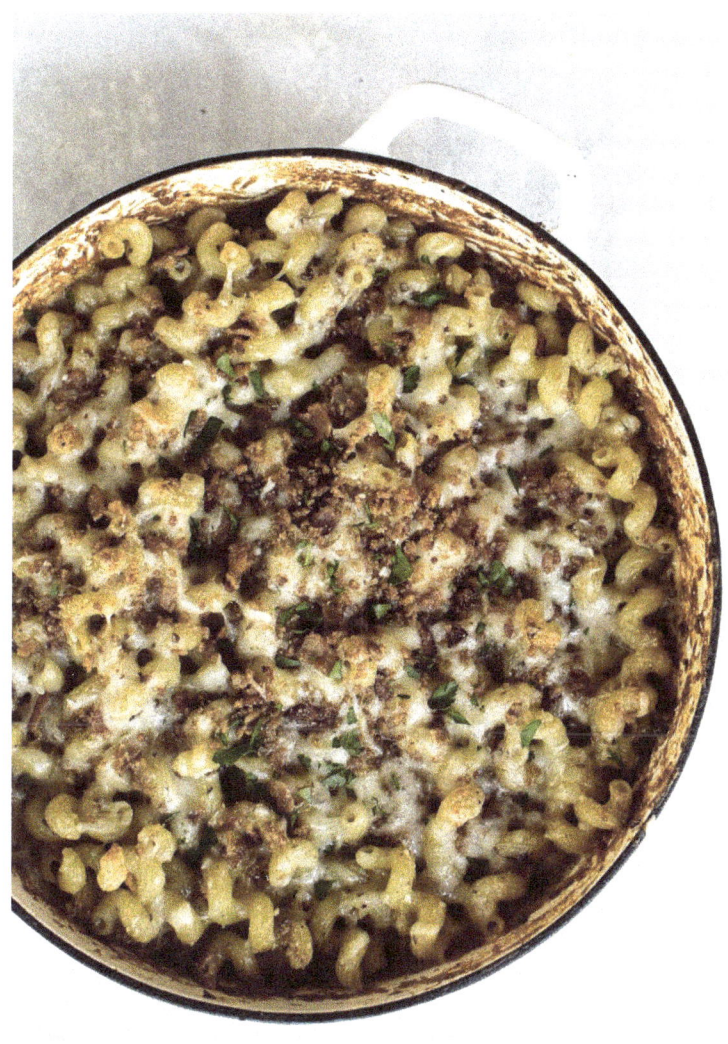

## Ingredients

1 red onion, medium chopped

¼ cup button mushrooms, drained

¼ cup cremini mushrooms

15 ounce can tomato sauce

28 ounce crushed tomatoes

4 tbsp. pesto

1 tsp. Italian seasoning

½ teaspoon salt

1/8 teaspoon black pepper

2 cups vegetable stock

8 ounces whole wheat elbow macaroni pasta uncooked

1 ½ cups Mozarella Cheese

Garnishing ingredients:

chopped green onions for serving

## Directions:

Put all of the ingredients except for pasta, cheese, and garnishing ingredients in your slow cooker. Combine and cover. Cook on high heat for 4 hours or low heat for 7 hours. Add the pasta and cooking on high heat for 18 minutes, or until pasta becomes al dente Add 1 cup of cheese and stir. Sprinkle with the remaining mozarella cheese and garnishing ingredients

# Papardelle Pasta and Oyster Mushroom and Vegan Chorizo

Ingredients

1 red onion, medium chopped

15 ounce tomato sauce

¼ cup oyster mushrooms, drained

28 ounce crushed tomatoes

1/4 cup vegan chorizos, coarsely chopped

1 tsp. dried thyme

½ teaspoon salt

1/8 teaspoon black pepper

2 cups vegetable stock

8 ounces pappardelle pasta uncooked

1 ½ cups Vegan Cheese (Tofu Based)

Garnishing ingredients:

chopped green onions for serving

**Directions:**

Put all of the ingredients except for pasta, vegan cheese, and garnishing ingredients in your slow cooker. Combine and cover. Cook on high heat for 4 hours or low heat for 7 hours. Add the

pasta and cooking on high heat for 18 minutes, or until pasta becomes al dente Add 1 cup of cheese and stir. Sprinkle with the remaining vegan cheese and garnishing ingredients

# Creamy Elbow Mac and Vegan Italian Sausage

**Ingredients**

1 red onion, medium chopped

1/4 cup vegan Italian sausage, coarsely chopped

1 cup oyster mushrooms

15 ounce can tomato sauce

28 ounce crushed tomatoes

4 tbsp. vegan cream cheese

1 tsp. herbs de Provence

½ teaspoon salt

1/8 teaspoon black pepper

2 cups vegetable stock

8 ounces whole wheat elbow macaroni pasta uncooked

1 ½ cups Vegan Cheese (Tofu Based)

Garnishing ingredients:

chopped green onions for serving

**Directions:**

Put all of the ingredients except for pasta, vegan cheese, and garnishing ingredients in your slow cooker. Combine and cover.

Cook on high heat for 4 hours or low heat for 7 hours. Add the pasta and cooking on high heat for 18 minutes, or until pasta becomes al dente Add 1 cup of cheese and stir. Sprinkle with the remaining vegan cheese and garnishing ingredients

# Pasta Shells with Tomato Sauce and Ricotta Cheese

## Ingredients

1 red onion, medium chopped

15 ounce can tomato sauce

28 ounce crushed tomatoes

3 ounces vegan mozzarella

1 tsp. Italian seasoning

½ teaspoon salt

1/8 teaspoon black pepper

2 cups vegetable stock

8 ounces pasta shells uncooked

1 ½ cups Ricotta Cheese

<u>Garnishing ingredients:</u>

chopped green onions for serving

## Directions:

Put all of the ingredients except for pasta, vegan cheese, and garnishing ingredients in your slow cooker. Combine and cover. Cook on high heat for 4 hours or low heat for 7 hours.

Add the pasta and cooking on high heat for 18 minutes, or until pasta becomes al dente Add 1 cup of Ricotta cheese and stir. Sprinkle with the remaining vegan cheese and garnishing ingredients

# Papardelle Pasta with Ricotta Cheese

## Ingredients

1 red onion, medium chopped

28 ounce crushed tomatoes

4 tbsp. pesto

4 tbsp. red pesto

1 tsp. Italian seasoning

½ teaspoon salt

1/8 teaspoon black pepper

2 cups vegetable stock

8 ounces pappardelle pasta uncooked

1 ½ cups Ricotta Cheese

<u>Garnishing ingredients:</u>

chopped green onions for serving

## Directions:

Put all of the ingredients except for pasta, vegan cheese, and garnishing ingredients in your slow cooker. Combine and cover. Cook on high heat for 4 hours or low heat for 7 hours.

Add the pasta and cooking on high heat for 18 minutes, or until pasta becomes al dente Add 1 cup of cheese and stir. Sprinkle with the remaining cheese and garnishing ingredients

# Lima Beans with Quinoa

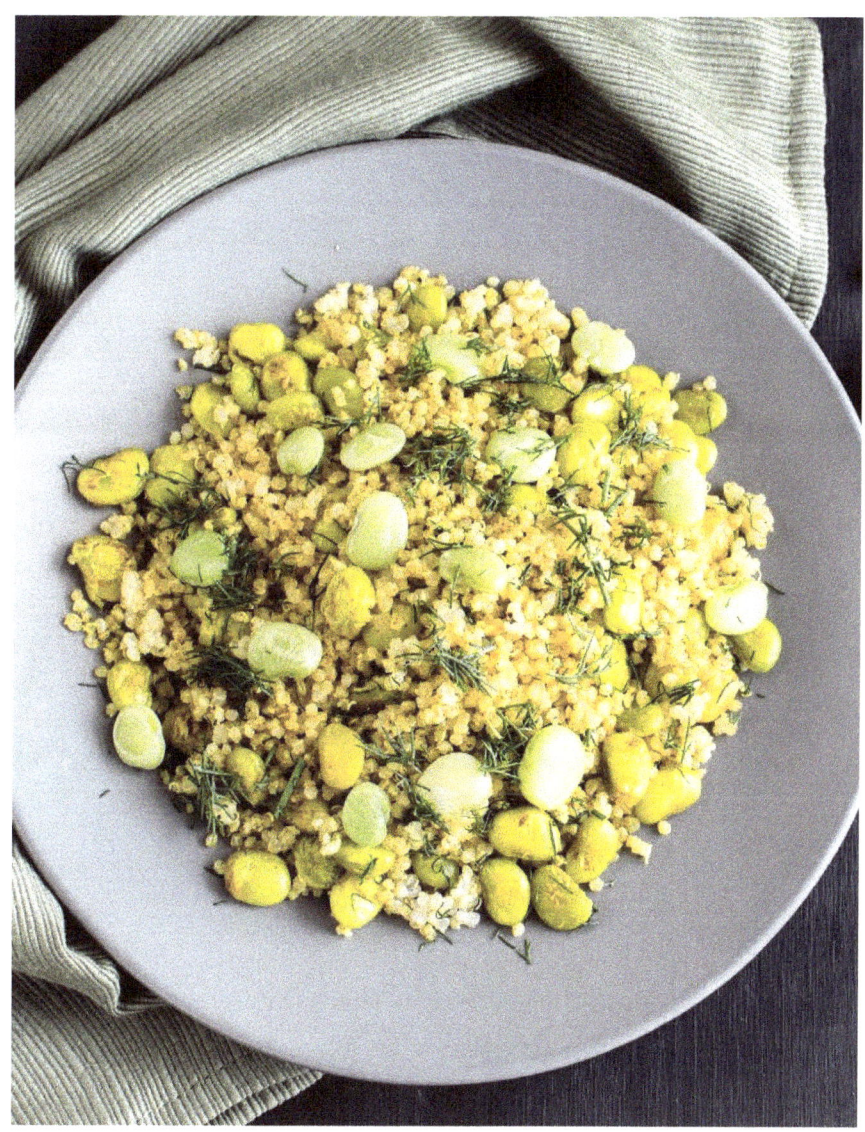

**Ingredients**

6 green bell peppers

1 cup uncooked quinoa, rinsed

1 14 ounce can garbanzo beans, rinsed and drained

1 14 ounce can lima beans

1 1/2 cups red enchilada sauce

2 tbsp. tomato paste

1 tsp. basil

1 tsp. Italian seasoning

1/2 teaspoon garlic powder

½ tsp. sea salt

1 1/2 cups shredded mozzarella cheese

Toppings:

cilantro, avocado.

Cut out the stems of the bell pepper.

**Directions:**

Take out the ribs and the seeds. Mix the quinoa, beans, enchilada sauce, spices, and 1 cup of the vegan cheese thoroughly. Fill each pepper with the quinoa and bean mixture. Pour half a cup water to the slow cooker. Place the peppers in the slow cooker (partially submerged in the water).

Cover and cook on low heat for 6 hours or high heat for 3 hours. Uncover and distribute the remaining vegan cheese over the tops of the peppers, and cover for a 4 to 5 minutes to melt the cheese. Top with cilantro & avocado

# Vegetarian Brown Rice Burrito Bowl

**Ingredients**

1 red onion, diced or thinly sliced

1 green bell pepper (I used yellow), diced

¼ cup gouda cheese, shredded

1 mild red chili, finely chopped

1 ½ cups black beans, drained

1 cup uncooked brown rice

1 ½ cups chopped tomatoes

½ cup water

1 tbsp chipotle hot sauce (or other favorite hot sauce)

1 tsp smoked paprika

1/2 tsp ground cumin

Sea salt

Black pepper

Toppings

fresh coriander (cilantro), chopped spring onions, sliced avocado, guacamole, etc.

**Directions:**

Combine all the burrito bowl ingredients (not toppings) in a slow cooker. Cook on low for 3 hours, or until the rice is cooked. Serve hot with coriander, spring onions, avocado and guacamole.

# Garbanzo Bean Burrito Bowl with Sun-dried Pesto

**Ingredients**

5 jalapeno peppers, diced

1 red onion, diced

1 mild red chili, finely chopped

1 ½ cups garbanzo beans, drained

1 cup uncooked red rice

1 ½ cups chopped tomatoes

½ cup water

4 tbsp. sun-dried tomato pesto

1 tsp. Italian seasoning

Sea salt

Black pepper

Toppings:

fresh coriander (cilantro), chopped spring onions, sliced avocado, guacamole, etc.

**Directions:**

Combine all the burrito bowl ingredients (not toppings) in a slow cooker. Cook on low for 3 hours, or until the rice is cooked. Serve hot with topping ingredients

# White Bean Vegetarian Burrito Bowl

## Ingredients

1 Anaheim pepper, diced

1 red onion, diced

1 mild red chili, finely chopped

1 1/2 cup white beans

1 cup uncooked white rice

1 1/2 cups chopped tomatoes

1/2 cup water

4 tbsp. pepper jack cheese, shredded

1 tsp. herbs de Provence

Sea salt

Black pepper

Toppings:

fresh coriander (cilantro), chopped spring onions, sliced avocado, guacamole, etc.

## Directions:

Combine all the burrito bowl ingredients (not toppings) in a slow cooker. Cook on low for 3 hours, or until the rice is cooked. Serve hot with topping ingredients

# Vegetarian Garbanzo Bean Burrito Bowl

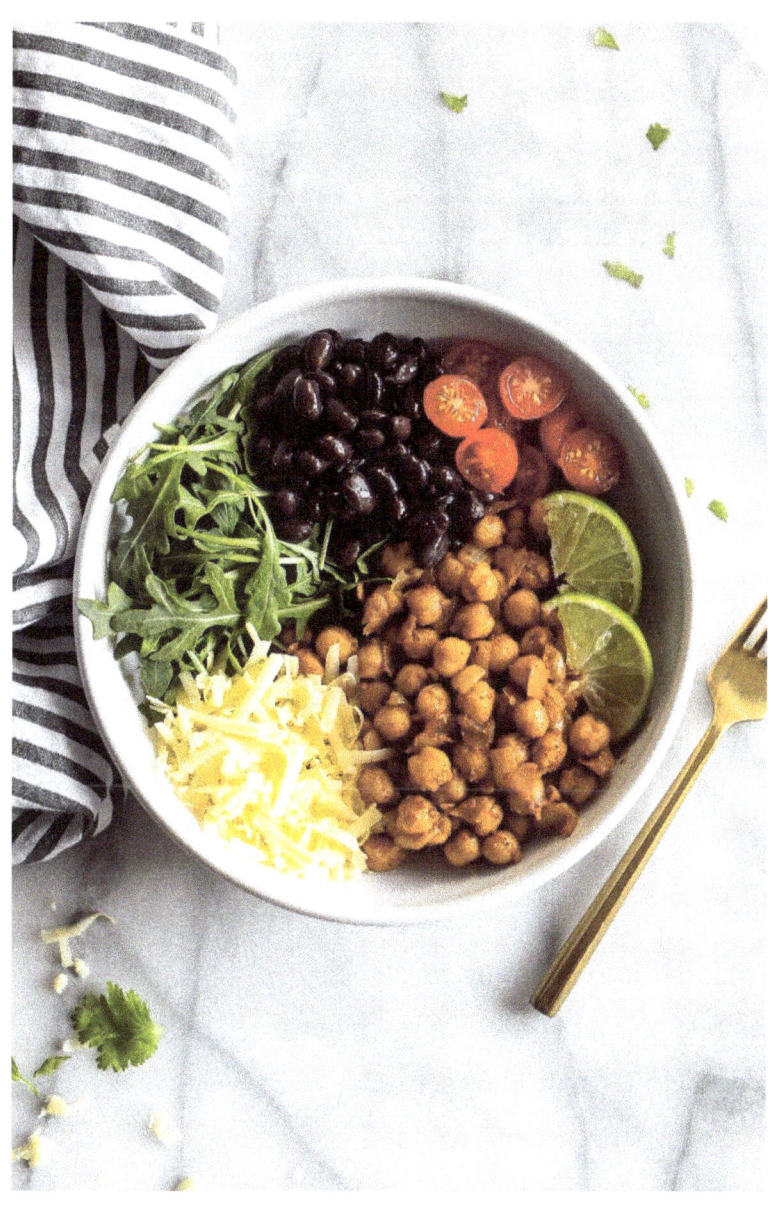

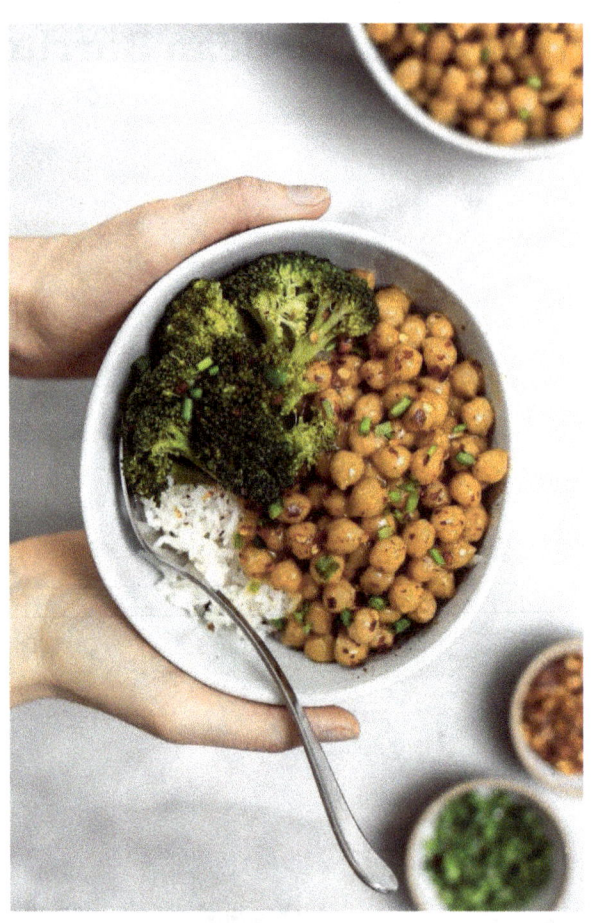

## Ingredients

1 red onion, diced or thinly sliced

1 green bell pepper (I used yellow), diced

1 mild red chili, finely chopped

1 ½ cups garbanzo beans, drained

1 cup uncooked red rice

1 ½ cups chopped San Marzano tomatoes

½ cup water

1 tbsp chipotle hot sauce (or other favorite hot sauce)

1 tsp smoked paprika

1/2 tsp ground cumin

Sea salt

Black pepper

Toppings:

fresh coriander (cilantro), chopped spring onions, sliced avocado, guacamole, etc.

**Directions:**

Combine all the burrito bowl ingredients (not toppings) in a slow cooker. Cook on low for 3 hours, or until the rice is cooked. Serve hot with topping ingredients

# White Bean and Ricotta Cheese Burrito Bowl

## Ingredients

1 ancho chili, diced

1 red onion, diced

1 mild red chili, finely chopped

1 1/2 cup white beans

1 cup uncooked white rice

1 1/2 cups chopped tomatoes

1/2 cup water

8 tbsp. Ricotta cheese, sliced thinly

1 tsp. herbs de Provence

Sea salt

Black pepper

Toppings:

fresh coriander (cilantro), chopped spring onions, sliced avocado, guacamole, etc.

**Directions:**

Combine all the burrito bowl ingredients (not toppings) in a slow cooker. Cook on low for 3 hours, or until the rice is cooked. Serve hot with topping ingredients

# Red Rice and Garbanzo Beans with Chimichurri Sauce

## Ingredients

5 Serrano peppers, diced

1 red onion, diced

1 mild red chili, finely chopped

1 ½ cups garbanzo beans, drained

1/2 cup vegan burger ( Brand: Beyond Meat Beyond Burger), crumbled

1 cup uncooked red rice

1 ½ cups chopped tomatoes

½ cup water

4 tbsp. chimichurri sauce

1/2 tsp. cayenne pepper

Sea salt

Black pepper

Toppings:

fresh coriander (cilantro), chopped spring onions, sliced avocado, guacamole, etc.

**Directions:**

Combine all the burrito bowl ingredients (not toppings) in a slow cooker. Cook on low for 3 hours, or until the rice is cooked. Serve hot with topping ingredients

# White Beans and Italian Sausage Burrito Bowl

## Ingredients

1 red onion, diced or thinly sliced

1 green bell pepper (I used yellow), diced

1 mild red chili, finely chopped

1 1/2 cup white beans

1/2 cup vegan Italian sausage, crumbled

1 cup uncooked white rice

1 1/2 cups chopped tomatoes

1/2 cup water

4 tbsp. pesto

1 tsp. Italian seasoning

Sea salt

Black pepper

Toppings:

fresh coriander (cilantro), chopped spring onions, sliced avocado, guacamole, etc.

**Directions:**

Combine all the burrito bowl ingredients (not toppings) in a slow cooker. Cook on low for 3 hours, or until the rice is cooked. Serve hot with topping ingredients

# Smoky Red Rice with Garbanzo Beans

## Ingredients

1 poblano chili, diced

1 red onion, diced

1 mild red chili, finely chopped

1/2 cup vegan burger ( Brand: Beyond Meat Beyond Burger), crumbled

1 ½ cups garbanzo beans, drained

1 cup uncooked red rice

1 ½ cups chopped tomatoes

½ cup water

4 tbsp. chimichurri sauce

1/2 tsp. cayenne pepper

Sea salt

Black pepper

Toppings:

fresh coriander (cilantro), chopped spring onions, sliced avocado, guacamole, etc.

**Directions:**

Combine all the burrito bowl ingredients (not toppings) in a slow cooker. Cook on low for 3 hours, or until the rice is cooked. Serve hot with topping ingredients

# Vegan Chorizo Burrito Bowl

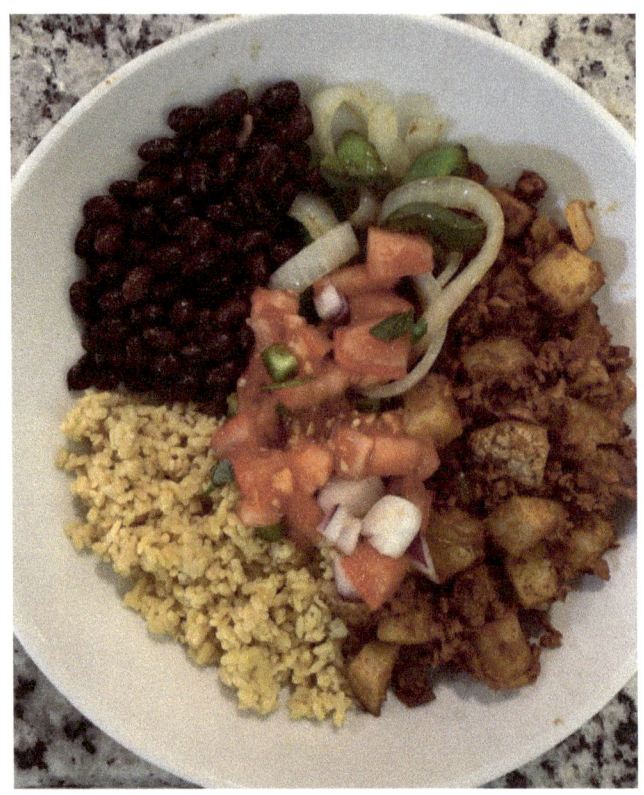

## Ingredients

1 ancho chili, diced

1 red onion, diced

1 mild red chili, finely chopped

1/2 cup vegan Chorizo ( Soyrizo), crumbled

1 cup uncooked white rice

1 1/2 cups chopped tomatoes

1/2 cup water

1/4 cup vegan chorizos, coarsely chopped

1 tsp. dried thyme

Sea salt

Black pepper

Toppings:

fresh coriander (cilantro), chopped spring onions, sliced avocado, guacamole, etc.

**Directions:**

Combine all the burrito bowl ingredients (not toppings) in a slow cooker. Cook on low for 3 hours, or until the rice is cooked. Serve hot with topping ingredients

# Chimichurri Vegan Chorizo Burrito Bowl

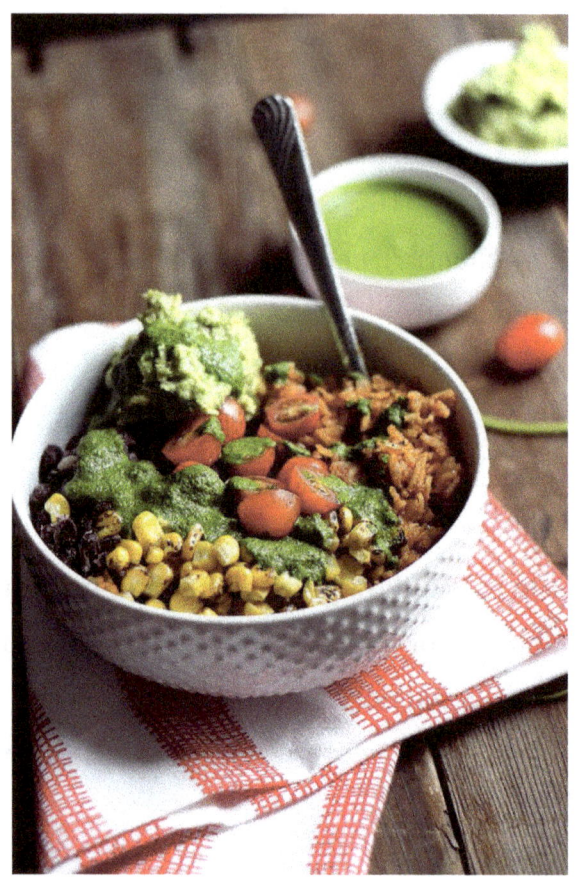

**Ingredients**

1 Anaheim pepper, diced

1 red onion, diced

1 mild red chili, finely chopped

1/2 cup vegan Chorizo ( Soyrizo), crumbled

1 cup uncooked red rice

1 ½ cups chopped tomatoes

½ cup water

4 tbsp. chimichurri sauce

1/2 tsp. cayenne pepper

Sea salt

Black pepper

Toppings:

fresh coriander (cilantro), chopped spring onions, sliced avocado, guacamole, etc.

**Directions:**

Combine all the burrito bowl ingredients (not toppings) in a slow cooker. Cook on low for 3 hours, or until the rice is cooked. Serve hot with topping ingredients

# Smoky White Bean & White Rice Burrito Bowl

**Ingredients**

1 red onion, diced or thinly sliced

1/2 cup meatless meatballs, crumbled

1 mild red chili, finely chopped

1 1/2 cup white beans

1 cup uncooked white rice

1 1/2 cups chopped tomatoes

1/2 cup water

1 tbsp chipotle hot sauce (or other favorite hot sauce)

1 tsp smoked paprika

1/2 tsp ground cumin

Sea salt

Black pepper

Toppings:

fresh coriander (cilantro), chopped spring onions, sliced avocado, guacamole, etc.

**Directions:**

Combine all the burrito bowl ingredients (not toppings) in a slow cooker. Cook on low for 3 hours, or until the rice is cooked. Serve hot with topping ingredients

# Red Rice with Vegan Chorizo and Tomatoes

## Ingredients

1 poblano chili, diced

1 red onion, diced

1/2 cup vegan Chorizo ( Soyrizo), crumbled

1 ½ cups garbanzo beans, drained

1 cup uncooked red rice

1 ½ cups chopped tomatoes

½ cup water

4 tbsp. chimichurri sauce

1/2 tsp. cayenne pepper

Sea salt

Black pepper

Toppings:

fresh coriander (cilantro), chopped spring onions, sliced avocado, guacamole, etc.

**Directions:**

Combine all the burrito bowl ingredients (not toppings) in a slow cooker. Cook on low for 3 hours, or until the rice is cooked. Serve hot with topping ingredients

# White Bean & Vegan Chorizo Burrito

**Ingredients**

1 ancho chili, diced

1 red onion, diced

1 mild red chili, finely chopped

1 1/2 cup white beans

1 cup uncooked white rice

1 1/2 cups chopped tomatoes

1/2 cup water

1/4 cup vegan chorizos, coarsely chopped

1/2 cup meatless meatballs, crumbled

1 tsp. dried thyme

Sea salt

Black pepper

Toppings:

fresh coriander (cilantro), chopped spring onions, sliced avocado, guacamole, etc.

**Directions:**

Combine all the burrito bowl ingredients (not toppings) in a slow cooker. Cook on low for 3 hours, or until the rice is cooked. Serve hot with topping ingredients

# Red Rice with Vegan Chorizo

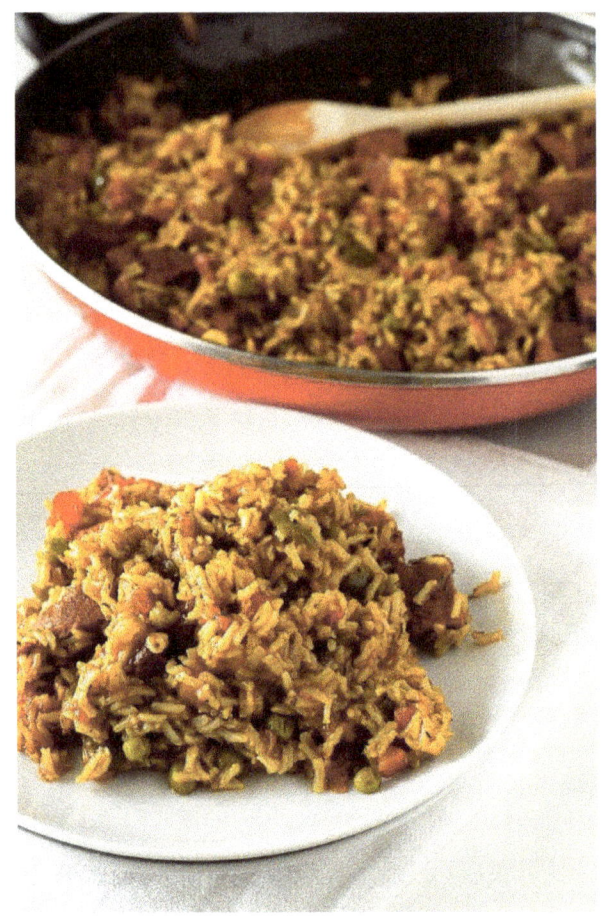

**Ingredients**

5 Serrano peppers, diced

1 red onion, diced

1/2 cup vegan Chorizo ( Soyrizo), crumbled

¼ cup capers, drained

1 cup uncooked red rice

1 ½ cups chopped tomatoes

½ cup water

4 tbsp. chimichurri sauce

1/2 tsp. cayenne pepper

Sea salt

Black pepper

Toppings:

fresh coriander (cilantro), chopped spring onions, sliced avocado, guacamole, etc.

**Directions:**

Combine all the burrito bowl ingredients (not toppings) in a slow cooker. Cook on low for 3 hours, or until the rice is cooked. Serve hot with topping ingredients

# Quinoa and Lima Bean Chili

## Ingredients

1 red onion, chopped

6 garlic cloves, minced

1 celery stalk, chopped

2 bell peppers, chopped

1 15 oz can diced tomatoes

4 cups vegetable broth

1 can water (I use the can of diced tomatoes to grab all the leftover flavor)

1 cup dried lentils

1 15 oz can Lima Beans

2 tablespoons chili powder

2 teaspoons cumin

1 tablespoon oregano

1/2 cup uncooked quinoa

1/4 teaspoon sea salt

**Directions:**

Put all of the ingredients into slow cooker. Cook on low for 8 hours or high for 4 hours. Serve with toppings such as shredded vegan cheese, avocado, green onion and cilantro

# Tangy Pesto Chili

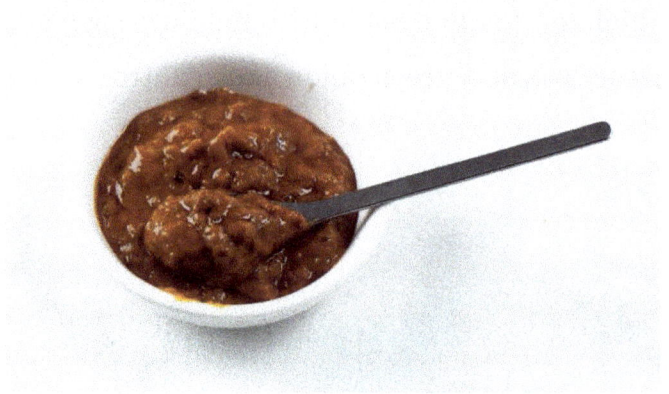

**Ingredients**

1 red onion, chopped

2 red onions

7 garlic cloves

1 ancho chili, minced

1 tbsp. lime juice

4 cups vegetable broth

1 can water (I use the can of diced tomatoes to grab all the leftover flavor)

8 oz. dried kidney

1 15 oz can White Beans

3 tablespoons pesto sauce

1 teaspoons dried basil, coarsely chopped

1 tsp. dried Italian seasoning

1/2 cup uncooked rice

1/4 teaspoon sea salt

**Directions:**

Put all of the ingredients into slow cooker. Cook on low for 8 hours or high for 4 hours. Serve with toppings such as shredded vegan cheese, avocado, green onion and cilantro

# Vegan Burger and Lentils

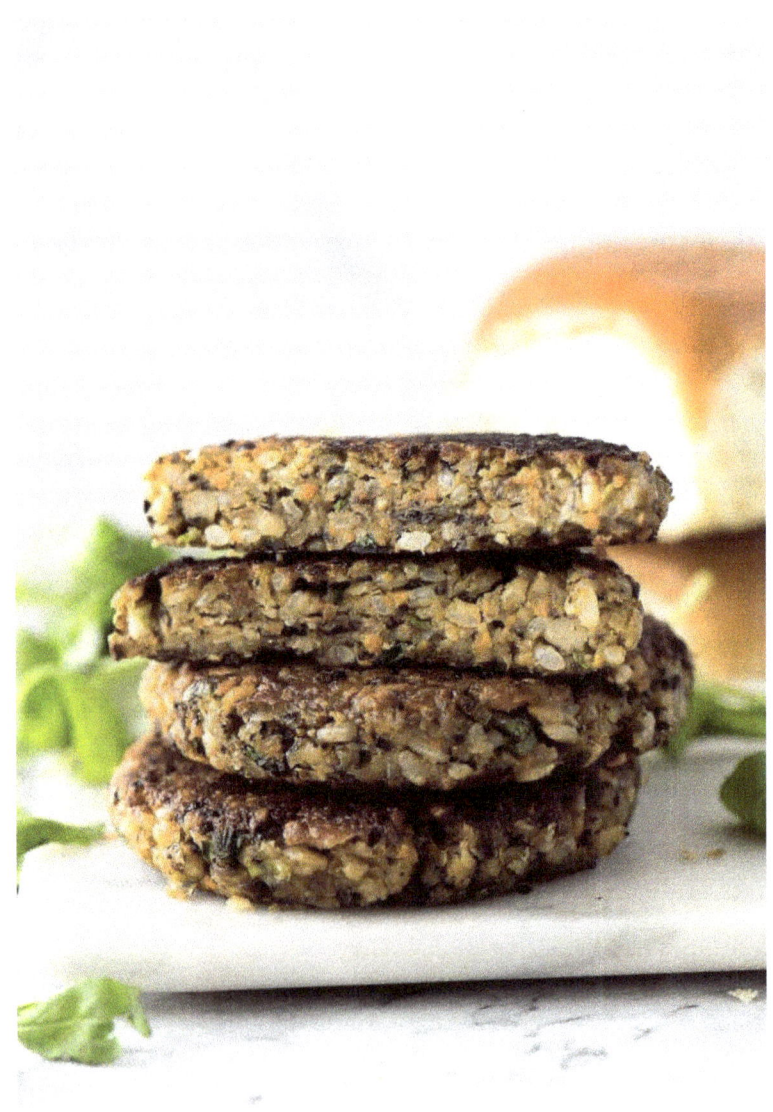

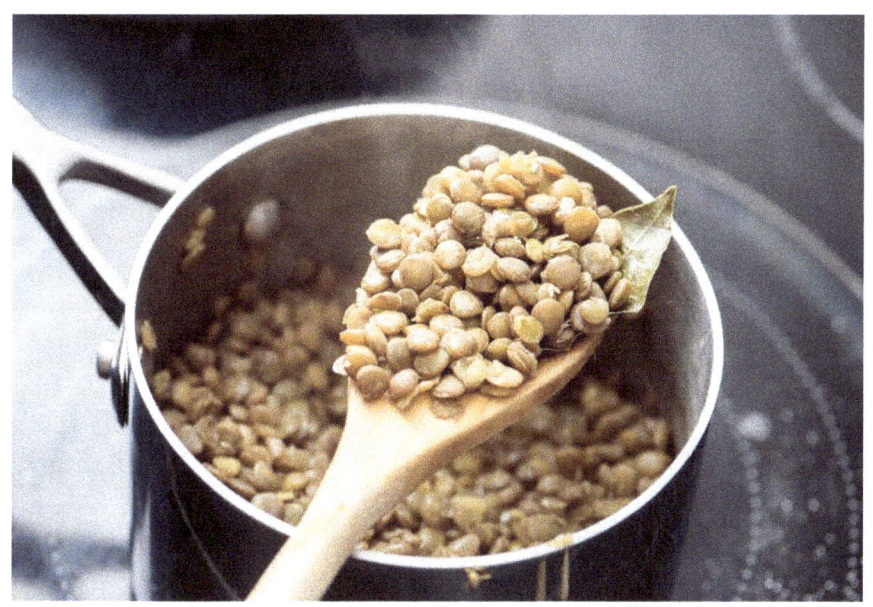

**Ingredients**

2 red onion, chopped

7 garlic cloves, minced

1 tsp. scallions, minced

1 tbsp. lemon juice

4 cups vegetable broth

1 can water (I use the can of diced tomatoes to grab all the leftover flavor)

8 oz. dried lentils

1/2 cup vegan burger ( Brand: Beyond Meat Beyond Burger), crumbled

2 tablespoons garlic powder

2 teaspoons onion powder

1 tablespoon herbs de Provence

1/2 cup uncooked red rice

1/4 teaspoon sea salt

**Directions:**

Put all of the ingredients into slow cooker. Cook on low for 8 hours or high for 4 hours. Serve with toppings such as shredded vegan cheese, avocado, green onion and cilantro

# Slow Cooked Thai Mung Beans and Black Rice

**Ingredients**

2 red onion, chopped

7 garlic cloves, minced

8 jalapeno peppers, minced

1 tbsp. lemon juice

4 cups vegetable broth

1 can water (I use the can of diced tomatoes to grab all the leftover flavor)

8 oz. dried mung beans

1 15 oz can button mushrooms

2 tablespoons garlic, minced

2 teaspoons chili powder

1 tablespoon Thai chili garlic paste

1/2 cup uncooked black rice

1/4 teaspoon sea salt

**Directions:**

Put all of the ingredients into slow cooker. Cook on low for 8 hours or high for 4 hours. Serve with toppings such as shredded vegan cheese, avocado, green onion and cilantro

# Quinoa with Beans

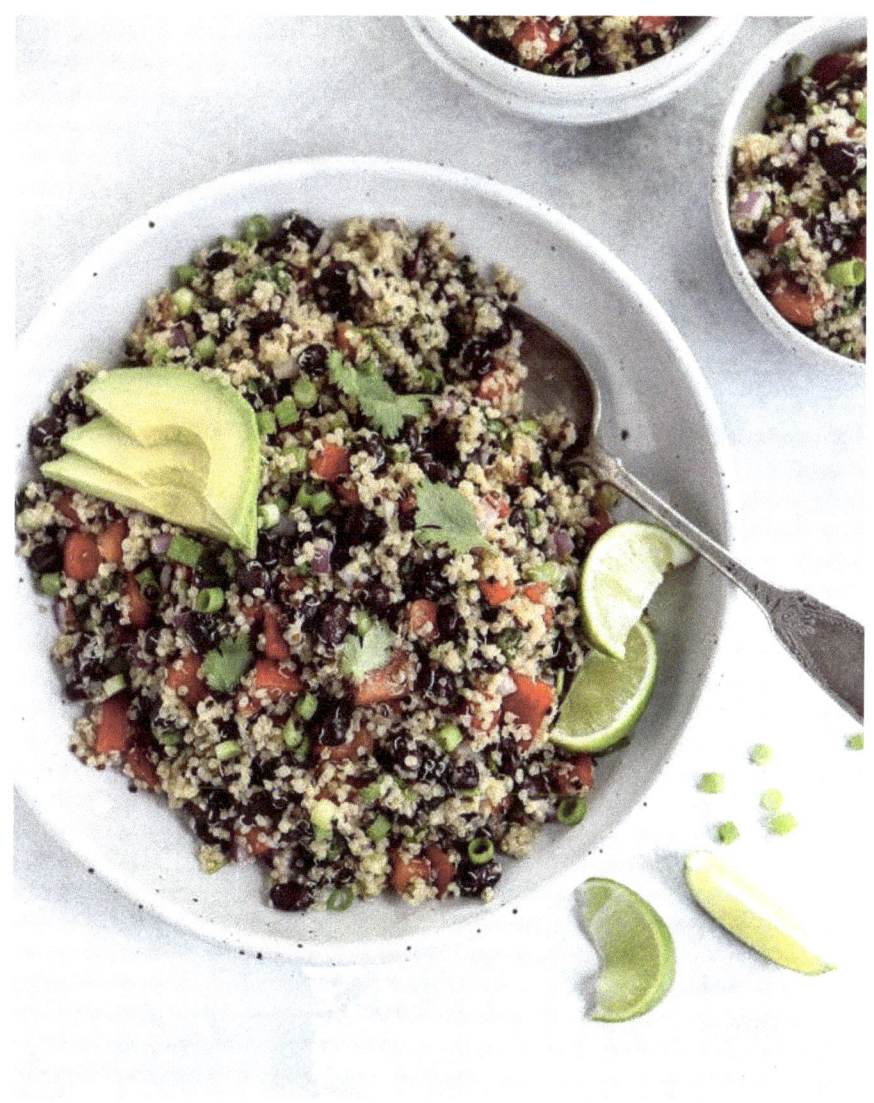

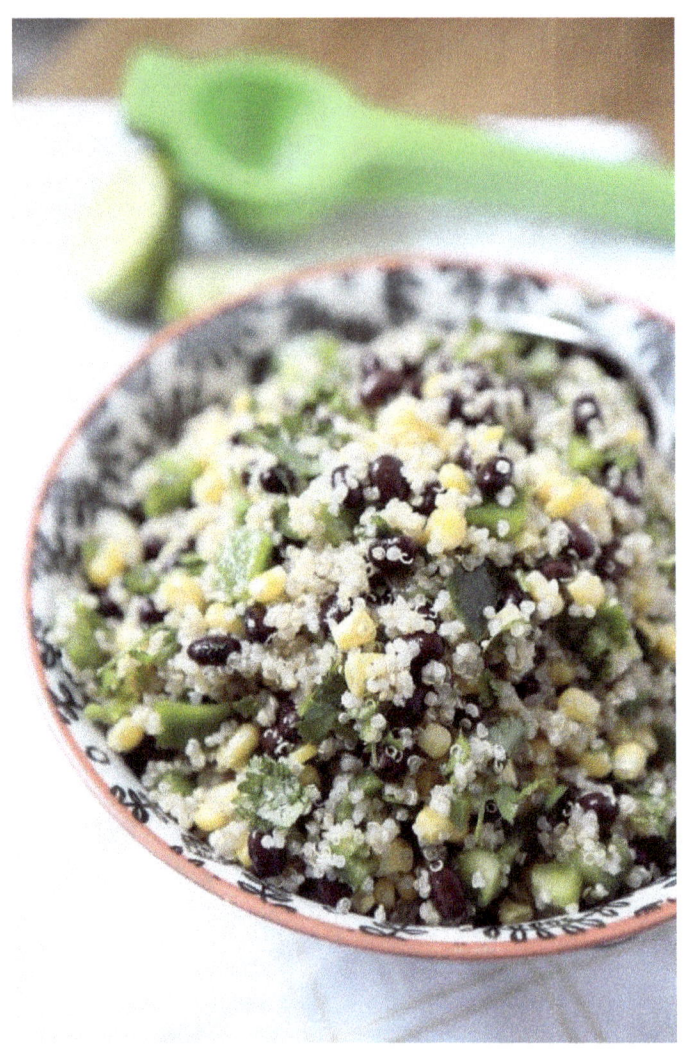

## Ingredients

1 red onion, chopped

6 garlic cloves, minced

1 celery stalk, chopped

2 bell peppers, chopped

1 15 oz can diced green tomatoes

4 cups vegetable broth

1 can water (I use the can of diced tomatoes to grab all the leftover flavor)

1 cup dried lentils

1 15 oz can Garbanzo Beans

2 tablespoons chili powder

2 teaspoons cumin

1 tablespoon oregano

1/2 cup uncooked quinoa

1/4 teaspoon sea salt

**Directions:**

Put all of the ingredients into slow cooker. Cook on low for 8 hours or high for 4 hours. Serve with toppings such as shredded vegan cheese, avocado, green onion and cilantro

# Smoky Brown Rice with Vegan Italian Sausage

**Ingredients**

2 red onion, chopped

7 garlic cloves, minced

8 jalapeno peppers, minced

1 tbsp. lemon juice

4 cups vegetable broth

1 can water (I use the can of diced tomatoes to grab all the leftover flavor)

8 oz. dried white beans

1/2 cup vegan Italian sausage, crumbled

2 tablespoons annatto seeds

2 teaspoons cumin

1 tsp. cayenne pepper

1/2 cup uncooked brown rice

1/4 teaspoon sea salt

**Directions:**

Put all of the ingredients into slow cooker. Cook on low for 8 hours or high for 4 hours. Serve with toppings such as shredded vegan cheese, avocado, green onion and cilantro

# Dried Black Beans and Quinoa in Pesto

**Ingredients**

1 red onion, chopped

2 red onions

7 garlic cloves

1 ancho chili, minced

1 tbsp. lime juice

4 cups vegetable broth

1 can water (I use the can of diced tomatoes to grab all the leftover flavor)

1/2 cup vegan Italian sausage, crumbled

1 15 oz can Black Beans

3 tablespoons pesto sauce

1 teaspoons dried basil, coarsely chopped

1 tsp. dried Italian seasoning

1/2 cup uncooked quinoa

1/4 teaspoon sea salt

**Directions:**

Put all of the ingredients into slow cooker. Cook on low for 8 hours or high for 4 hours. Serve with toppings such as shredded vegan cheese, avocado, green onion and cilantro

# Vegetarian Meatballs and Quinoa

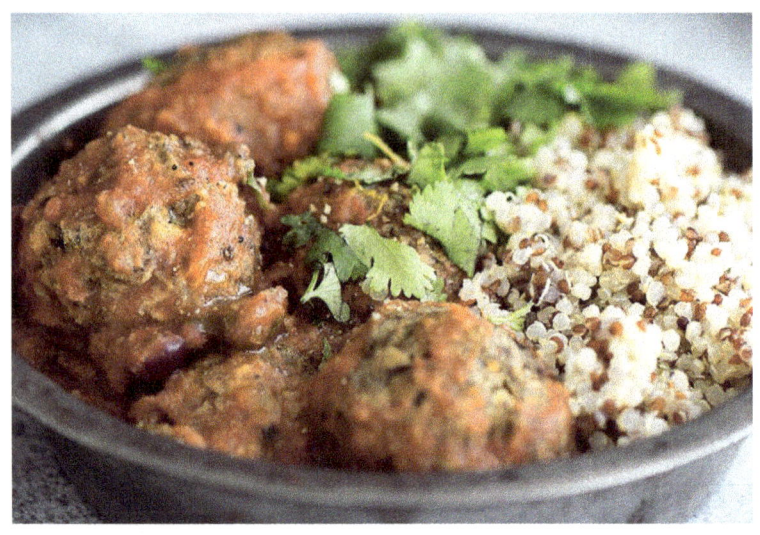

**Ingredients**

2 red onion, chopped

7 garlic cloves, minced

8 jalapeno peppers, minced

1 tbsp. lemon juice

4 cups vegetable broth

1 can water (I use the can of diced tomatoes to grab all the leftover flavor)

1 cup dried lentils

1/2 cup meatless meatballs, crumbled

2 tablespoons chili powder

2 teaspoons cumin

1 tablespoon oregano

1/2 cup uncooked quinoa

1/4 teaspoon sea salt

**Directions:**

Put all of the ingredients into slow cooker. Cook on low for 8 hours or high for 4 hours. Serve with toppings such as shredded vegan cheese, avocado, green onion and cilantro

# Slow Cooked Thai Black Rice with Mung Beans

## Ingredients

2 red onions, chopped

7 garlic cloves, minced

1 tsp. scallions, minced

1 tbsp. lemon juice

1 15 oz can diced green tomatoes

4 cups vegetable broth

1 can water (I use the can of diced tomatoes to grab all the leftover flavor)

8 oz. dried mung beans

1 15 oz can Black Beans

2 tablespoons garlic, minced

2 teaspoons chili powder

1 tablespoon Thai chili garlic paste

1/2 cup uncooked black rice

1/4 teaspoon sea salt

**Directions:**

Put all of the ingredients into slow cooker. Cook on low for 8 hours or high for 4 hours. Serve with toppings such as shredded vegan cheese, avocado, green onion and cilantro

# Red Rice and Vegetarian Meat Sausage with Jalapeno Pepper

## Ingredients

2 red onion, chopped

7 garlic cloves, minced

8 jalapeno peppers, minced

1 tbsp. lemon juice

4 cups vegetable broth

1 can water (I use the can of diced tomatoes to grab all the leftover flavor)

8 oz. dried lentils

1/2 cup vegetarian grain meat sausages, crumbled

2 tablespoons garlic powder

2 teaspoons onion powder

1 tablespoon herbs de Provence

1/2 cup uncooked red rice

1/4 teaspoon sea salt

**Directions:**

Put all of the ingredients into slow cooker. Cook on low for 8 hours or high for 4 hours. Serve with toppings such as shredded vegan cheese, avocado, green onion and cilantro

# Spicy Brown Rice with Vegan Chorizo

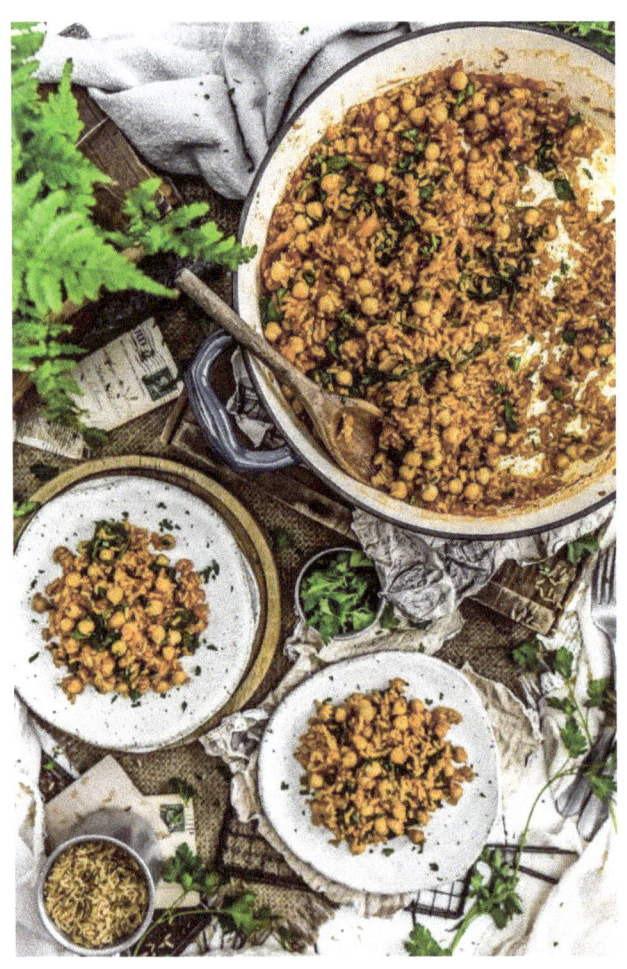

## Ingredients

1 red onion, chopped

6 garlic cloves, minced

1 celery stalk, chopped

2 bell peppers, chopped

1 15 oz can diced tomatoes

4 cups vegetable broth

1 can water (I use the can of diced tomatoes to grab all the leftover flavor)

1/2 cup vegan Chorizo ( Soyrizo), crumbled

1 15 oz can Black Beans

2 tablespoons annatto seeds

2 teaspoons cumin

1 tsp. cayenne pepper

1/2 cup uncooked brown rice

1/4 teaspoon sea salt

**Directions:**

Put all of the ingredients into slow cooker. Cook on low for 8 hours or high for 4 hours. Serve with toppings such as shredded vegan cheese, avocado, green onion and cilantro

# Kidney Beans & Button Mushrooms with Pesto Sauce

## Ingredients

2 red onions

7 garlic cloves

1 ancho chili, minced

1 tbsp. lime juice

4 cups vegetable broth

1 can water (I use the can of diced tomatoes to grab all the leftover flavor)

8 oz. dried kidney beans

1 15 oz can button mushrooms

3 tablespoons pesto sauce

1 teaspoons dried basil, coarsely chopped

1 tsp. dried Italian seasoning

1/2 cup uncooked rice

1/4 teaspoon sea salt

**Directions:**

Put all of the ingredients into slow cooker. Cook on low for 8 hours or high for 4 hours. Serve with toppings such as shredded vegan cheese, avocado, green onion and cilantro

www.ingramcontent.com/pod-product-compliance
Lightning Source LLC
Chambersburg PA
CBHW070735030426
42336CB00013B/1982